# Chronic Fatigue

# Syndrome

I0407503

# And

# Me

# Table of Contents

2nd Edition
Published by BDS Distributors
Copyright 2018 by BDS Distributors

# Introduction

I first came down with Chronic Fatigue Syndrome back in 1990. I was hit hard with the illness. I went to all different types of doctors and had every test you can think of done. Everything always came out good. I was medicated for Major Depression, it helped somewhat but still did not do the trick. After many years the illness did get better. Last year 2016 my sister had a heart attack. I had to get rid of all her cats and her apartment. This put a big load on me. At the same time, I had several losses due to death. I started to get tired a lot and next thing I knew it I was back to where I was years ago. I remember the day it all hit me suddenly. I was visiting my sister at the nursing home and I watched her walk with the therapist. She looked like she was 80 years old, but she was only 61. Suddenly, I got very tired and fatigue. It was an hour drive home and after I left her I had to park and take a nap before heading back home.

I did a lot of research recently not only to help myself but hopefully it will help someone else.

CFS's is not a new illness. It has been around for years. Not only women can get it but also men.

The best advice I can give you is take your time and read the book. You can also do research on your own.

Take one day at a time and sometimes one second at a time. That is how I get by each day

Best wishes

Bruce Dolan Smith

# Chapter 1

## Definition

Let us start off with the definition of Chronic Fatigue Syndrome. It is exactly as is reads, "Chronic Fatigue". To me Chronic Fatigue is just more than being tired all the time. In the United States the illness is called Chronic Fatigue Syndrome (CFS) and overseas it is known as Myalgic Encephalomyelitis (ME). With CFS a person may get some rest or sleep, but they do not feel refreshed when they wake up. As far as myself I must rest or take frequent naps throughout the day. I do not "per say" sleep I just rest my eyes. My best part of the day right now is first thing in the morning. In the afternoon is when my body starts to shut down for the day. I try not to plan too much on one given day. Also, when I schedule any appointments if I can I schedule them all first thing in the morning.

The illness affects several systems in the body at the same time. It affects the immune system, the nervous system, and the endocrine system. Any illness that affect one system being each cell share the same receptor will affect the other two systems.

According to the Center for Disease Control and Prevention. Chronic fatigue syndrome, or CFS, is a debilitating and complex disorder characterized by profound fatigue that does not improved by bed rest and that may be worsened by physical or mental activity. Symptoms affect several body systems and may include weakness, muscle pain, impaired memory and or mental concentration, and insomnia, which can result in reduced participation in daily activities.

The CDC looks at the individual. If they have had severe chronic fatigue for more than 6 months which it is not due to heavy exertion or other medical conditions which is found in other illness with severe fatigue. These other conditions need to be ruled out after the necessary tests have been done. If all test comes out to be normal then more than likely they have, "Chronic Fatigue Syndrome."

# Chapter 2

## What causes Chronic Fatigue Syndrome?

As of right now researchers and doctors have not been able to come up with once single cause of CFS. There are some theories that a wide variety of viruses could cause it such as: Epstein Barr virus, herpes viruses and the retrovirus XMRV. Other theories are that some people inherited the virus, an interaction between neurotransmitters and hormones and that it may be caused by some type of trauma that has happened in the person's life. Also, there are other illness which could cause CFS. As of right now I have been thru many different kinds of test. The only thing that is helping me now is keeping active as much as I can, I do get a lot of rest during the day.

I know last year I had a lot of losses due to death. Before this I was feeling ok however feeling very fatigue at the end of the day. My sister had a heart attack which I was under a lot of stress. I had to empty her apartment and find homes for her cats. The following summer my fatigue worsened. Then I had some friends die. It got to the point where I could not do anything. All I did was rest and sleep. As time went by with me not being active I started to gain weight. I also was in and out of the hospital for high blood pressure, stomach problems. While I was in the hospital I had a lot of test done. My heart was good however I had some problems with my stomach. I had a procedure done recently on my stomach which opened my intestine more, so my food would digest better. I am also Bi Polar which I think my depression came back not realizing it. I have to admit I am doing somewhat better now. I switched psychiatrist and moved to another apartment. My new psychiatrist changed my medications which started to help. It is winter still here in New Jersey so once the weather gets warmer I am going to start walking each day only little at a time. I am also going to buy a treadmill which will help me also. The key thing with CFS is keep active as much as you can even if you only do a little at a time. I keep my mind active which keeps my mind from the illness. I listen to music, watch TV, and write.

As doctors and researchers try to find the cause of CFS I am not sure if they will really find what causes this mysterious illness.

It is January 19,2018.  My Chronic Fatigue

Syndrome got worse again.  I am very tired and fatigue

all day.  I have muscle spasms, pain all in my body,

numbness and tingling feeling.  I do not know why the

illness came back to me.  All I do all day is rest, listen

to music and watch T.V.  I go to bed real early and I

am awake a lot of times thru out the night.  I keep track

of my steps that I take each day on my cell phone.

Yesterday I think I over did it.  I walked around 2400

steps.  It really is not a lot of steps of the average person

but for someone with CFS I think it is a lot.  I am

paying for it today.  I am very exhausted and cannot

sleep.  I figured I would do some writing to help make

me tired, so I can fall asleep.

People rated on a percentage rate of what they think cause their illness:

- Immune/viral factors

  100%

- Stress                                65%

- Genetic/Hereditary factors            43%

- Toxic exposure                        43%

- Allergies                             37%

- Emotional Trauma                      37%

- Physical Trauma                       28%

- Diet                                  28%

Below are several easy-to-use coping techniques. Read each statement and on a scale of 1 to 7 showing where you would locate yourself on the scale:

1. My motivation is lower when I am fatigue

Completely disagree                    Completely

Agree

1    2    3    4    5    6    7

2. Exercise brings on my fatigue

Completely disagree

Completely Agree

1    2    3    4    5    6    7

3.  I am easily fatigue

Completely disagree

Completely Agree

    1    2    3    4    5    6    7

4.  Fatigue interferes with my physical functioning

Completely disagree

    Completely Agree

    1    2    3    4    5    6    7

5.  Fatigue causes frequent problems for me

Completely Disagree           Completely

Agree

1    2    3    4    5    6    7

6. My fatigue prevents sustained physical functioning

Completely disagree

Completely Agree

1    2    3    4    5    6    7

7. Fatigue interferes with carrying out certain duties and responsibilities.

Completely disagree

Completely Agree

1    2    3    4    5    6    7

8. Fatigue is among my three most disabling symptoms.

Completely disagree

Completely Agree

1    2    3    4    5    6    7

9. Fatigue interferes with my work, family, or social life.

Completely disagree

Completely Agree

1    2    3    4    5    6    7

How to Score: Add up your numerical answers and divide them by nine. Scores which range from 6.0 and 7.0 indicates a severe, and persistent fatigue. Average of 3.0 indicates a healthy adult. For a range of 4.5 to

6.5 highly signifies elevation over depressed patients.

# Chapter 3

## Understanding CFS

Chronic Fatigue Syndrome can be a long-term disorder. It effects a lot of the systems in the body. The most debilitating symptom being fatigue. Other symptoms can be poor sleep, pain, and confusion. A person may develop depression because of being sick so long and so profound. Also, a person can develop such emotional problems such as anxiety, irritability, and grief. I know myself right now seems like I am going thru a type of grief process because I miss the old things I use to be able to do. I will see people on TV that are older than me and think boy look how healthy they are. It can and will affect people's lives because there are a lot of adjustment one has to make. It is hard because we have to try to control the symptoms such as pain, fatigue and whatever one suffers from. It can cause a financial burden on a family because CFS can be so server where a person cannot work. I am on disability right now and I know I cannot work at all. It feels like a loss because there are just things we use to be able to do and just cannot any more. It can cause stress on the family because the things you use to be able to do, someone else has to do it for you. These are all adjustments that one has to make and accept. Some people's illness may not be so bad as another's. The key thing is keep a positive outlook. There are others that are affected by the illness where they are home bound and cannot go out at all.

# Chapter 4

## Diagnosing and Testing

Doctors should consider ordering all test that are necessary to rule out illness that may be like the symptoms a person may have with CFS. All routine test such as complete blood count, urinalysis and a liver function test should be given as part of the initial examination.

Recently I once again developed chronic fatigue. Being it has been so long that I was sick with the illness my doctor order a lot of tests. To rule out any brain injury I had a SCAT scan done, a complete blood work up to rule out leukemia, MS, kidney disease, liver disease, thyroid disease, infections such as Lyme, and autoimmune diseases. Because of my age and that I am a diabetic I had a complete work up done on my heart.

All my tests came out to be normal. I can remember years ago, when I first came down with CFS I have a lot of different symptoms than I do today. Basically, I am just very fatigue all the time and have some weird headaches from time to time.

.

# Chapter 5

## The Beginning of a Long and Serious Illness

I was first diagnosed with CFS in 1990. At the time, I lived in Florida and we had problems with mosquitos carrying Encephalitis. I can remember we were told not to out at night unless we had to. If we did go out, we should wear long sleeve shirts and pants. Some of the games at night were cancelled. This did not scare me, I went out to the pool in our apartment complex swimming and just wearing a pair of shorts. Well sad to say but this lead to a very serious illness.

It was not much longer after we had the Encephalitis scare I had to go to the hospital. My mother and my sister went to Disney World in Orlando. I could have gone also but I just was not feeling all that good. On my way into work I was starting to sweat and felt very fatigue. I got into work and as time went by the worse I was feeling. I just had to go back home. I told my boss that I was leaving. I decided to go to the emergency room to get checked out. The closer I got to the hospital the worse I was feeling. I just could not take it any longer. I stopped in a gas station and told the attendant to call for the ambulance. I had to put the air conditioner on because it started to feel as if I was going to black out. It seemed like hours for the squad to get to me, but it was only five or ten minutes. Once they got me in the back of the rescue squad I started to feel a little bit better. Well once I got into the emergency room the doctor had all sorts of test done. The doctor told me that all my tests were normal, and he sent me home.  As soon as I got off the bed in the ER I stood up and my legs just felt like rubber.  I got home, and I still was not feeling well at all.  My friend's father stayed with me until my mother and sister got back from Disney World.  I could not work for a few weeks.  All I did was rest and did not much at all.

The medical doctor I was seeing at the time told me it was depression, but I knew it was much more than that.  I continued to see him for a little while but as time went by I still has not feeling well.  I felt as though he was not helping me at all.  I went to see a neurologist. He was great, this doctor listened to me and what symptoms I was having.  I had to have all sorts of tests done again.  A lot of them came back normal.  He diagnoses me as having Post Encephalitis

# Chapter 6

## My first Hospitalization

As time went by I was not getting any better. I called my doctor up and told his secretary that I was suicidal. She got ahold of the doctor, right away he called me on the phone. He told me the best thing for me at the time was to be admitted to the hospital. Once again, I had to have a lot of test done. Most came back normal however my arsenic level was very high. I had to think for a minute, doesn't arsenic come from rat poison. I said to myself no this could not be, are my mother and sister trying to kill me? I was in for about a week when the doctor was ready to discharge me. I felt the same way as the way I came into the hospital. I talked to the doctor and he had me transferred to their behavior ward. This was the first time I was ever in a psych ward. I went in to the groups they had during the day. Different people were telling their own story. As I listen to each one the more it was sounding like me, I was having the same symptoms. This time they were calling it anxiety or panic attacks. The first part of my illness was Post Encephalitis and the second was problems with anxiety. I was in for about 7 days. When I went home I was feeling a little bit better. Finally, after about a week home from the hospital I was able to go back to work.

I had a very good paying job however I was under a lot of stress. My bosses wanted me to quit but I did not give in. Finally, I did quit. I just could not continue working there.  It took some take, after a while I started

to feel better.

# Chapter 7

## Managing with Chronic Fatigue Syndrome

How does a person manage with having Chronic Fatigue? Well for myself right now I try not to schedule any appoints in the afternoon. I make all my appointments if I can first thing in the morning. I figure I may have about 30 minutes' worth of energy before I need to rest. I am going to bed early right now. It is not like other illness where you stay in bed for a couple of days and you are over it. This is just the opposite with CFS, no matter how much rest you may get you still feel very fatigue.

I have a regular medical doctor who sees me, also I have a psychiatrist and a therapist to help me. The therapist helps me out, so I can have a person to tell how I feel each day. It is good to talk about all problems a person may have. I changed psychiatrist, I found one that accepts Medicare who specializes in Chronic Fatigue Syndrome. He changed some medications and added some new medications. I'm beginning to feel somewhat better.

I have been thinking on why did I get hit with CFS again. Well I have been under a lot of stress this past year with my sister having a heart attack. I had to pack up her entire apartment and get rid of her 7 cats. Also, at the same time I was working on starting my own taxi cab business. So, with all of that it just took a toll on me. Funny is at the time I did not think I was under stress.

The hardest part of my day right now is in the afternoon. Right now, it is summer, and it has been very hot lately. The heat bothers me just like everyone else, only it affects me even more. I have been feeling somewhat better. I try to do whatever I need to first thing in the morning. It is a good thing that I am on disability right now because there is no way I can work right now.

Last month I went to my doctor which led me to the hospital emergency room. I had all sorts of blood test done. All test came out normal. Every once in while especially when the disease is present I always have test done. Right now, I have to be very careful that I do not overdo and at the same time I do not do the opposite, that is sit around and do nothing. I have to say this time around with CFS I am not getting nearly as much symptoms as I was back in the 90's. The only thing I have that is affecting me is like the disease is called, "Chronic Fatigue." Along with the fatigue I have a little problem with anxiety. The anxiety is not as bad as it was years ago. I do not need to take any medication for the anxiety.

I can remember when I first came down with the illness I was worse than I am now. There would be times where I was in bed for days on end. I was not active at all and because of this my muscles started to get weak, especially in my legs. At times, I would have to take my mother food shopping and when I did I had to use the electric carts because of my legs being so weak. In order for me to get my leg muscles back again I would go walking at night with my mother around our apartment complex. It would take time but eventually I got the use of my legs back.

Because of the illness, I ended up having to quit my job. The job I had at the time was very stressful and this did not help me at all. I was kind of relieved after quitting. I eventually got a job as a security guard at night. This was an easy job and it was a lot cooler at night than it was during the day. I worked from 8pm to 4am three days a week. There would be times that I would have to stop working because of my illness. I go back into the hospital once again. This time I would go to the psych hospital. There was and still is not much that can be done for CFS but just rest. By me going in the hospital it more less forced me to rest. The security guard job I had at the time was very good to me. They understood and took me back when I was well enough to work again.  Sad to say but this cycle went on for a few years.

As your symptoms arise you will have to be strong.  As I have mentioned earlier I had a lot of different symptoms.  I had a lot of test and all of them can out normal.  Some days I feel like the illness is going to take over me however I remind myself about the tests and what the doctors said to me.

I try to keep active as much as I can.  I just moved in my new apartment.  This keeps me busy. I had a lot of boxes to unpack.  Today is Thursday March 16, 2017.  All of the moving is finished.  I just have a few things to unpack and I will be done with the move.

What helps me get by during the day and helps me to go to sleep is listening to self-hypnosis relaxing videos on YouTube.  This helps me a lot to fall asleep.

I listen to them during the day sometimes also to help

me get a good rest.

# Chapter 8

## Symptoms

There are a lot of different symptoms that comes along with having CFS. That is why it is very important to have tests done to rule out any other illness that it can be. The symptoms that you can have are fatigue, memory loss, sleep disturbance, unrefreshing sleep, flu like symptoms, muscle and joint ache, numbness or tingling sensations, depression, anxiety, panic attacks, muscle weakness, Abdominal pain, diarrhea, nausea, gas, irritable bowel, Heart palpitations and Chest pain. There are other symptoms that you may have. It is a good idea to find a doctor in your area that specializes in Chronic Fatigue Syndrome. Four symptoms that are usually accompanied with CFS are:

- Fatigue can be explained as a very deep exhaustion. It can be brought on low levels of activity or for no apparent reason. Fatigue can be caused by over activity, poor sleep, deconditioning, stress, and poor eating habits.

- Pain can be in the joints or overall pain all over. It feels as though you got over by a truck. Pain can be brought on and intensified by over activity, poor sleep, anxiety, stress, and changes in the weather.

In order to diagnose CFS your doctor will want to rule out other illness that has the same symptoms Chronic Fatigue Syndrome. Below are just a few illnesses that mimic CFS:

- The Flu: The flu has many CFS like symptoms. However, the flu does not last six or more months.

- Fibromyalgia: Fibromyalgia is just like CFS both of them are very hard to diagnose. The difference between the two is that Fibromyalgia's primary symptom is having muscle and joint pain and CFS first symptom you must be fatigue.

- Lyme disease: Both diseases have overlapping symptoms.

- Hormonal disorders: for this your thyroid needs to be checked.

- Sleep disorders: Anything that interfere with having a good night sleep can be the cause of Chronic Fatigue Syndrome. I myself have sleep apnea and I use the CPAP machine. Even if I a m resting for the day I will put the mask on.

- Depression and other mental disorders: Some mental illnesses can cause chronic fatigue. Also, some medications to treat a mental illness can cause fatigue.

- Eating disorders: A proper diet can help if you have CFS

- Lupus: Symptoms The symptoms of Lupus has about the same as Chronic Fatigue Syndrome.

- Obesity: Having even just an extra ten pounds can make you feel fatigue and tired

- Alcohol and other drugs can cause all types of side effects. One of them is fatigue.

Your doctor should rule out the above illness to be sure you do not have any of them. Before going to your doctor, it would be a good idea to write down on a piece of paper they symptoms you are having. This will be a good start to help your doctor to determine if you have CFS. Below is a list of the most common tests should be given to a person who is suspected of having CFS:

- ✓ Complete Blood Count (CBC)and blood chemistry
- ✓ Thyroid function study
- ✓ Sedimentation rate
- ✓ Urinalysis
- ✓ CT Scan and or MRI

There are questionnaires could help to determine if

you have Chronic Fatigue Syndrome.

# Chapter 9

## Learn how to pace yourself

Living with Chronic Fatigue Syndrome we need to learn how to pace ourselves. I realize it can be hard at times just sitting around and not being able to do much. It is ok to plan activities to do but just do not take on too much in one day. Try to limit your activity to maybe one or two per day. As time goes by you can increase your activity to more than just two. This will help you keep somewhat busy during the day time and not to burn out. Trust me I know first-hand what it is like to overdo yourself. Try to do things when you are at you best. Be sure to take many rest periods as you need to. This will also help you not to overdo it. Should you overdo it either physically or mentally can cause your illness to ether come back or get worse. If you notice that your symptoms are coming back, then this is telling your body you are over doing it. If there are just those things that should get done and you are not able to do it ask for help. There is nothing wrong with asking for help. I am sure people around you will be more than happy to lend a helping hand. Another good tool to use is a daily and weekly schedule. If you plan something for one day and do not get it done go ahead and put it on the schedule for the next day. I remember one day I over did it. I was at a Ham fest which is like a flea market for Ham Radio Operators. I did a lot of walking and started to feel it at the end of the day. I was not over my illness yet and this just sent be back even further. For the one day of over doing it I had to rest completely for three days.

The most important thing with any illness whether it is physical or mental is acceptance. Once you come to that big word of acceptance you can then move on. Years ago, when I first got diagnosed as being Bi Polar I was not willing to accept my illness as being mental. I was going to all sorts of doctors and having many unnecessary tests done. Once I was able to accept my illness as being mental that was when I was on the road of recovery. Chronic Fatigue Syndrome is the same. Sure, we all need to have the proper and unnecessary tests done from time to time. It is when everything is ruled out then we can relax.

Also, what can help tremendously is treat the symptoms you are having at the time. I take over the counter pain medications to treat all pain I have. The other problem I have is not being able to fall asleep. I am on some medications for my mental illness which also helps me to sleep well. If you also have problems sleeping and not taking anything for it, I would suggest asking your doctor what you can take. Finally, what can help us all with this mysterious illness is relaxation and stress reduction strategies. Try to listen to smoothing music you like. There are many ways to relax. By listening to music, you like helps get your mind from negative thinking. Also, what is very important to do is try to keep positive. It may be hard at times with being fatigue daily. The more positive you are the more positive you are going to feel.

I often think of how I felt before or I may be watching a movie and I think to myself boy what is it like to be able to walk on that beach. This is when hopelessness comes in to play. What I have to do is think positive. One day I will be over my storm and will be able to walk on that beach. For now, yes, I have some good minutes and I am able to rest when I want. I am very fortunate that my rent is reasonable, and my car is paid for. I think what would be best for all of us is make a gratitude list. Write down what we do have, even if it seems to be small. Try to keep a journal of how you are feeling, the symptoms you are having and the duration. You should see an improvement over time. Even if it is just a small improvement, small is better than nothing. I know for myself for example today was a very hard day for me. I could not sleep at all last night and I had a few things that just had to get done. Now it is 9 pm as I am writing this, and I am very tired. My mind is being occupied but the thing is once I stop writing my body will suddenly crash. But at least I did get some things done and did not over do it.

I think most of us with CFS have to sleep or take frequent naps during the day, even if we are having a good day. Sometimes I feel guilty taking many rest breaks during the day. This is how I get by each day. Now the past few nights I have been having difficulty falling asleep. Perhaps I may be getting to much rest during the day however like I said I have to do this right now.

I have noticed if I overdo it when I stop doing whatever activity I feel my body and mind crashing.

However, it is very important to keep active without over doing yourself.

# Chapter 10

## Listen to Your Body

Having CFS we must listen to what our body is telling us. As I mentioned in a previous chapter write down a daily schedule. Do not over book yourself. This is only setting you up for failure. It is ok to just to two things in one day. There may be a day where you are just not up to do anything. This also is ok. The key thing is do not overdo it. On the other hand, do not do the opposite and that is under do yourself. Even if it means just making yourself lunch, taking a shower, or just watching TV. The more you do the better. It will get your mind off the illness. This does not mean to run the marathon. It just means to keep active the best you can. I have problems when at the end of the day I really feel fatigue. This means my body is telling me to sit back and relax the rest of the day. I find a good movie on TV or just listen to music. By me listening to music this totally relaxes my body and mind. Make personal rules for yourself. Write down on a piece of paper what your limitations are. Some days you may have to adjust your limitations. There may be a day where you feel great. Be careful on days like this that you do not overdo it. Just listen to what your body is telling you and take frequent breaks. Take as many breaks as you have to. When I say, you need to rest I mean complete rest. This means none of the following: exercising, no visitors, telephone calls (turn your phone off), computers. Anything that may count as an activity. You want to try to rest your entire body along with your mind. Some smoothing music should help rest both mind and body. By doing all this I have mentioned should help you to better listen to what your body is telling you.

If you can relax as little as 20 minutes a day you will find it has powerful health-inducing effects. By relaxing at least 20 minutes a day you will find the following:

- Dissipate the accumulated tensions of the day

- Reduce your anxiety and worry

- Create a sense of well-being

- Help you cope with stress

- Give you a sense of control over symptoms as well as your reactions to them

- Improve the restfulness of your sleep

There are other important physical benefits is you would take time out to rest at least 20 minutes a day. Studies have shown there are improvements in immune functioning.

Because of the severity of my illness I have to rest a lot of times a day. I find it very helpful when I listen to the YouTube videos on relaxation.

# Chapter 11

## Making adjustments in your life

Living with CFS we all need to make adjustments in our life style. Chronic Fatigue Syndrome is a real disease. If you are working, you may want to consider going out on disability for a while. The more rest you get the better. The time frame on getting better or over the illness can vary from person to person. I have done some research on CFS and there are people that are bed ridden. I am fortunate that I am not one of them. That is why I insist that we who are living with CFS need to make some changes in our life style. I take some medications for Bi Polar at bed time. They also help me sleep, right now I take the medications around 4pm instead of 9pm. It does take several hours to take effect. This enables to give my body the proper rest it needs. I also take frequent and long rest periods during the day. If I have any appointments I have to keep I try to schedule them before 1pm. Sure, there are some days that I am more fatigue than others. This just means I need to rest more on those days. I look back and try to figure out how I came down with CFS again. I look back at the past two years and I can see where I was under a lot of stress. I do not have nearly as many of the symptoms as I did back in the 90's. basically, I just do not have the energy or at the end of the day I am very fatigue. I am hoping that with a lot of rest and cut back on stress in my life I will once again overcome this illness. We all have stress in our lives I realize but it is how we deal with it. I can get into that subject but that will just be another book. Best advice I can give you and can give myself is make the necessary cut back on your life style. Keep active but learn do not overdo it.

We all have things that must be done daily. The best way is to first make a list of what needs to be done. If there are some things that you know you cannot do at all ask someone to help you. I am sure there is a family member or friend that would be willing to do this for you. Today if you have a computer there are a lot of things that you can do online such as: pay your bills, go shopping. In my area, there is a grocery store that you and go shopping on line and they will even deliver it to you. This will be very helpful since food shopping can be very tiresome. It is even out of the question for us with CFS to do. Last week I made a mistake and went to do some food shopping with a friend. Well needless to say I paid for it the next four days. You can even ask churches in your area if they have volunteers whose mission is to help shut-ins.

There may be sometimes you do not want to talk of the phone. All you should do is either screen your calls or just turn the phone on silence. You can let your friends know that after a certain time you do not want a call at all. I am sure they will understand.

Be careful of what type of TV shows you watch. You may not realize it however any type of show such as stressful news programs, movies or specials on murder, thrillers, horror moves. We all know in today's times watching the news can be very stressful. The key thing is to try to eliminate any and all stressors that you can. Try to watch comedies, mysteries, old movies. You want to do these things because it does not take any energy to do and at the same time it will get keep your mind occupied.

If you are able to take a short walk outside. This will help to keep the muscles in tune. I cannot stress enough the key thing is do not over do it. If one day you planned on taking a walk and just do not feel up to it by all means stay in.

There are several ways to help you make adjustments in your life. One thing that does not help anyone with Chronic Fatigue Syndrome is stress. Stress just makes your symptoms worse. Here are just a few ways that will help you with stress. Use meditation, biofeedback, deep breathing, hypnosis, relaxation tapes, listen to music, if you can go for a short walk. They are just a few ways I am sure you can find some more ways to combat the stress in your life.

No matter what illness we have can cause stress. The key thing is keep your mind off your illness. You want to try to keep your mind busy and your mind from any distractions. Some of the ways you can do this is watch TV, listen to music, turn the lights off and turn your phone off. By doing these things will help you keep your mind from your illness. The other ways to keep your mind busy are reading a good book, watch fish in a tank, knitting. The men can go fishing and any other ways to keep your mind distracted. When you think of what to do think of things that require no effort of your end.

# Chapter 12

## Is there treatment for CFS?

I have been told by some of the doctors that I saw for illness that there is no cure. That did not stop me in doing research on CFS. I realize everyone is different. What may help me my not help you. Here are some of the treatments that you can try: Herbal remedies, massage, manual manipulation techniques, nutritional supplements and stress reduction methods such as meditation and bio feedback.

On October 24, 2011 researchers in Norway experimented on 30 people who had CFS. They were given a biologic drug that effects the immune system. The drug that was given to the 30 patients was Rituxan. It works by affection the immune cells called B-cell.

For the study half was given infusion of saline solution as a placebo and the other half was given two infusions of rituximab which was given two weeks apart. Rituximab is used for treatment of non-Hodgkin's lymphoma, chronic lymphocytic leukemia rheumatoid arthritis.  67% patients and 13% saw a moderate reduction in being fatigue.  Out of the 30 patients three that was given the rituximab continued to be symptom free 2 ½ years later. The question is with the 30 patients that did this study only three of them remain symptom free 2 1/2 years later would you still like to try the drug rituximab.

The National Institute for Health and Care Excellence and a group of doctors did a study on some people whom had CFS.  They recommended just two treatments, graded exercise therapy (GET) and (CBT) cognitive behavioral therapy. GET is a program that patients increase exercises in small amounts daily. Exercises include stretching, range of motion contractions and extensions. These exercises are done only a few minutes each day. Each day the exercises are increased a little at a time. Also, CBT is usually included with the program. Both the doctors and patients did not like the GET program because they feared by exercising may cause a relapse. While at the same time other doctors believed by exercising a little each day will help the patients improve over time. Instead they paced themselves and listened to what their bodies was telling them trying not to do too much, wary of pushing themselves thinking that their illness may get worse. What I am doing right now is pacing myself. I realize that I must be careful that I do not overdo and then on the other hand that I do just the opposite. While I am being very careful on what I do I am also seeing a therapist to help me mentally. I am also walking every other day at our mall where I live.

There are other alternative treatments to help reduce the severity of specific symptoms. When patients took more of a nutritional supplement and included a non-drug therapy such as dieting, rest, taking frequent naps, and modified their activity helped reduce their symptoms. I rest as much as I have to and take many naps during the day. A lot of times I will listen to music to help get my mind off the illness. Below are some of the alternative therapy that can be used:

- To relive pain acupressure and acupuncture, chiropractic, massage tens, reflexology can be used.

- To help relive anxiety and Stress Reduction: Biofeedback, Meditation, Hypnosis, Yoga, Visualization, and Guided Imagery. There may be other alternative treatments that can help manage the symptoms a person may have.

- Some medications may also help with the pain associated with CFS. You can try over the counter pain medications.

- Individual Psychiatric or Psychological therapy: by having a one-on-one mental health therapy secession my help. This part of the treatment plan can help the person by venting how he or she is feeling. This can help if a person has symptoms of depression or anxiety. I know myself I am seeing a psychiatrist to help me with the illness.

I went and made an appointment with a psychiatrist. I am presently seeing one in my area, but she does not seem to be helping me at all. Even though I told her the symptoms I have been having she did not make any changes in my medication. I switched doctors. The doctor I am seeing now is both a psychiatrist and neurologist. He did make some changes in my medications and added a few new ones. It has been about two weeks now since I have seen him, and I am already feeling somewhat better. It seems like my mood is more positive and I can do a little more than I was doing before. I still get tired during the day, but it does not seem to me so bad. I still rest a lot and try not to overdo it but a least I have noticed some improvements.

Home treatment for CFS is the most important part of the treatment. Some good ideas you may want to try are:

- Take advantage of the times you do have more energy. This is the time to do the things you really need to do.

- Keep a journal for a week. Write down when you do have energy and then write down the time your energy level changes.

- You may be able to plan your day easier by knowing the time of day you are at your best.

- Try not to overdo it when you do have more energy. Remember if you overdo it you may pay for it later.

- Make adjustments in your sleep habits. Go to sleep only when you are tired and feel sleepy. Wake up the same time each morning.

- If you are awake for more than fifteen minutes, then it is time for you to get up. Leave the bedroom. Do something quite until you are sleepy again. Then try to go back to sleep.

- Do not drink any caffeine or alcohol before going to bed. Both are stimulants and they will just keep you awake.

- Be sure the bedroom is at a good temperature. It is a good idea to make it as dark as possible. You will find this will help you sleep much better.

- Take naps when you need to during the day. Keep them short about 20 to 60 minutes at a time. Try not to take a nap in the late afternoon.

- Exercise a little each day. You may want to start out with stretching. When you can go for short walks. Swimming is the best exercise. Remember do not over do it. If you are very tired the next day, then cut back the amount of time you are exercising.

# Chapter 13

## Putting together a good Treatment Plan

Being CFS is such a complicated illness with symptoms vary day from day it is a good idea to have a good treatment plan lined up.  Below is an example of a good treatment plan you can have in place:

- Medications: These includes painkillers, antidepressants, antianxiety mediations. Any type of medication that can help with the symptoms you are having at the time.

- Individual psychiatric or psychological therapy: This means by you having a one on one with both your psychiatrist and therapist. They both help you to monitor your symptoms. The psychiatrist will prescribe medications he or she may feel will help elevate some of the symptoms you are experiencing. While your therapist can help listen to the symptoms you are having and determine the best treatment plan to have.

- Alternative Care: This is by taking natural herbs and supplements. Other alternative care treatment are massage, yoga, and mediation.

This can help relieve the stress that you may have. I myself like to listen to YouTube videos on mediation and talk down to help you sleep. This helps me out a lot. Perhaps you can try it.

- Managing your life and sleep: Many people with CFS has sleep problems. The key is to balance out your sleep schedule to your waking life. To get the proper sleep, you should not sleep much during the day. If you sleep too much this will throw your sleep schedule off balance. So, it is important to balance out your waking and sleeping life.

- Eating Healthy: It is important that you eat healthy meals, so your body gets the proper nutritional. If you eat healthy you should find you will have more energy and less fatigue.

- Exercising: This may sound crazy telling someone with CFS they should exercise. When I say exercise, I do not mean to go for a mile jog or walk for an hour. I just mean to walk as much as you can without over doing it. You need to pace yourself. My cell phone has a step counter in it. I try to take 2000 steps a day which is not really much at all. I am increasing my steps I take a little at a time. I am not quite up to 2000 steps yet. If you find it hard to walk outside, then just walk inside your house or apartment. Go for small walks until you feel your body can do. I cannot emphasize enough Pace yourself do not overdo it otherwise you will just be at the beginning again.

- Getting rid of stress: Granted we all have stress in some form or another the key thing is how we deal with it. Talk to someone about your problems this will help reduce the amount of stress you are carrying. The best way to deal with stress is to confront it right away and take care of whatever needs to be done. You will find if you are under a lot of stress your symptoms will get worse.

# Chapter 14

## Anxiety and CFS

One of the symptoms you may have is anxiety. The best way to deal with it is to speak to your doctor. There are several different medications that may help you.

Another good way to help control your anxiety is to have a good therapist.  He or she can listen to you and it will help you get anything that is bothering you.  There are also some self-help groups or centers out there for you to go to.  Sure, I understand that it is hard having chronic fatigue all the time and I understand that you do not really want to go out.  The best time for you to try these groups is when you are at your best.  For me I am at my best first thing in the morning.  Any time after 1pm my body tells me to rest.  So, what I do is try to make all appointments in the morning.  There is a very good Self-Help Center by me however it is open in the afternoons only.  Because afternoons are when I am at my worst I cannot go.  I do see a very good therapist however.  She helps me out a lot by like I said above is just by listening to me. She also comes up with some very good suggestions.

See if there is a group for people with CFS in your area. Unfortunately, there is not any in my area. You may want to ask your doctor or check with the hospital in your area to see if they know of any type of groups that my help you.

Chapter 15

Coping with having Chronic Fatigue

How does one cope with having CFS or any other serious illness. First off, all you need to avoid physical stress. When having Chronic Fatigue Syndrome, you need to listen to your body. Be prepared your body is not the same as it used to be. Should you be just exercising or simply walking can set off a chain reaction that can leave you in bed for days. I know just recently I started to walk at our mall in town. Well that is ok however I over did it. I went every day for about a week. I paid for it the next days to follow. We all need to set boundaries when it comes to having Chronic Fatigue Syndrome. Below are just a few things you should try to avoid:

- *Avoid extremes of temperature*
- *Avoid strain*
- *Maintain a regular meal*

- *Maintain a regular sleep schedule*

Minimize Psychological and Emotional Stress By having unnecessary stress can make the illness worse. I realize we all have stress in our lives however it is how we deal with it. If you can find someone you can talk to. Perhaps a good friend, relative, clergy or a family member. The key thing is talk to someone about your problems. What happens is if you do not deal with your problems you will be like a pressure cooker and eventually blow up.

There are some stressful situations that just cannot be avoid, such as a loss of your job, death of a friend for family member, an accident and more. There are also those minor stressful situations that also cannot be avoided such as a doctor's appointment, medical tests or even as minor as a visit from a family member or friend. Both stressful situations can produce symptoms. Some of these situations cannot be avoided but all you have to do is to learn how to deal with these situations as they happen. Try to put all your appointments on a calendar so they do not suddenly appear. This should help the situations not to be so stressful. The key with living with CFS is try to eliminate all your stressors.

When you make your weekly list of things you have to do learn to priorities your list. As I mentioned earlier if you do not get something done on Monday then just add it to Tuesdays list.

Learn to say no. There may be times when a family member or friend will want you to do something. In your mind, you know it will be just too much for you to do. You do not want to overdo yourself because it will just end you up back at the beginning of your illness. The more you say NO to someone the easier it will get. I am sure they will understand.

You may start a project and have very good intensions of completing it, but your illness creeps up on you again. It is ok to put it aside to finish once you feel better. Do not stress yourself because you did not get it done. Sometimes there are those tasks that must get done. Do not be afraid and ask someone for help. I am sure a friend or family member will be more than happy to help you.

Try to go out when your body tells you that you can. Investigate what types of self-help groups are in your area. This is what helps me when I can go to our self-help center in town because I listen to other people's experience with their illness by doing this also keeps

my mind busy and off my own illness.

A good way that can help you cope is keep a journal,

do research on CFS and write about it. You can learn

about the illness by researching it. Once you know

more about Chronic Fatigue Syndrome the better you

will be able to cope with it. Also, you may find some

treatments that you may want to try

## Chapter 16

What does Chronic Fatigue Syndrome feel like?

Chronic Fatigue Syndrome is different from person

to person. For example, I feel exhausted by the end of

the day. I am extremely tried through the day. There

are days when I am so tired that I am not able to do

anything but rest. Yes, I do have some good days if that is what you what to call good days. I take naps frequently and even by doing that after my nap is over I am still very tired. I feel like I am a prisoner in my own body. I cannot drive right now because of the CFS. My friend has my car right now and is what I call chauffeuring me around for the time being. Because of being tired and exhausted at the same time does interfere with a person's life and work.

A good idea is to write down on a piece of paper all of the symptoms you are having, sometimes you may forget something. Keep a journal of how you are feeling. Keep track of your sleep, pain, fatigue and whatever else you are experiencing.

# Chapter 17

## Relationships and CFS

Having relationships, no matter who they are they can be your best friend, a family member, or your spouse. Sometimes people do not understand the illness we have. This can make it hard on both parties.

It may be a good idea if you ask them to do some research on the illness. I should tell you if they are truly your friend or they truly love you they will do the research. This is a good idea, so they can understand a little of what you are going thru. I realize it is hard on not only on them, but it is hard also on us who have the illness. Living with Chronic Fatigue Syndrome is hard because most of the time you may not want to go out. Being fatigue all the time means just that, (fatigue.) Be prepared that you may lose some friend because of the illness. This just means that they were not truly your friend. Here you will find out who your friends really are.

Having CFS attaches stigma to those who are ill. The people who do not understand and thinks it is all up in your head therefore in the beginning of this chapter I write it is a good idea for them to do research on Chronic Fatigue Syndrome. The more your friends or family understand the illness the better they will be able to help you.

It might be harder if you are single and not dating any one your potential boy/girlfriend may find it hard to accept because an illness like CFS is very complex. I know with myself it is especially hard on making new friends. People in general may not believe CFS is a real disease. Some people may think that you are just faking it, or you are just tired. What they do not know is yes, I am tired, but it is different than when a normal person is tired. There are a lot more symptoms that goes along with the illness. We have to remember we are not here to please people we are here to get by one day at a time.

If you are a parent you may find it lot harder trying to keep up with your children. There may be a lot of times where you will have to say no to them. If you do just the opposite, you will find it will catch up with you. This will just make your illness worse than it already is. After a while by saying no the easier it will be.

You will want to tell your children about your illness, so they will not worry and think you are going to die. The more they know the more your children can cope with the disease. You may find that instead of them asking you to do something they will do things on their own.

# Chapter 18

## Work and Disability

You may find it hard to work having CFS. I remember when I first got sick back in 1990 I struggled every day going in to work. Finally, I just had to quit my job. I was lucky because I was living at home with my mother and sister. I considered collecting Social Security Disability. It took me 1 ½ years to finally get approved for SSD. I was turned down twice and then the last time I had to get a lawyer. I do not know what I would have done if I lived on my own. There are some of you reading this book saying the same thing. It is not worth the aggravation to continue working. I realize we all need money to survive but it does not help if you cannot work at all. You may be able to work part time on your job.  Explain to your employer that you are sick and cannot work full time right now you may have to get a letter from your doctor.  Depends on how sick you are whether I would suggest you working at all right now.  I know when I first got sick I could not work at all finally accouple of years I was able to work part time.  There were times when I would have to take a few months off.  I had a very understanding employer that would let me come back when I was able to.  I am still on disability thank God because I am haunted with CFS once again.  At this present time, I am not able to work at all.

# Chapter 19

## My experience having Chronic Fatigue Syndrome

Living with CFS can be hard some days. Years ago, when I first came down with it I had all sorts of symptoms. I had server headaches, sweats, muscle weakness and more. Today I should say I only have a few symptoms. I get very fatigue during the day and my legs get weak. Right now, I have bronchitis and fighting the flu this just makes me feel even worse. I rest a lot during the day and try to keep myself somewhat busy. I figure for every 30 minutes of activity I rest about an hour right now. I do not keep going although. Once my body tells me it is time to stop for the day then I stop. There are some days that I just think I'm dying or there is something serious wrong with me. I did have all sorts of medical tests done recently and everything came back normal. Sometimes I wonder if I am going to get over this hump I am in. Years ago, I was a lot younger and it did take some time. There for a while my legs were very weak, so I would go for walks with my mother around our apartment complex in the evening. My legs are very weak now, so I have to start walking a little each day. The only problem I have like I just mentioned is I am sick with the flu. I do keep my mind occupied by watching movies. There are sometimes I have to give my mind a break and I listen to music. This is good because it passes the time a way and it keeps my mind off my illness. I went food shopping with a friend of mine today and I used their electric cart. It made my shopping a lot easier and I did not get so fatigue like I would have if I walked. If you are able to get out do not overdo it and use the electric carts the stores provide.

# Chapter 20

## Learning about Chronic Fatigue Syndrome

Chronic Fatigue Syndrome is like mental illness there is no one test that can say yes you have CFS. If you break your arm you can have an x-ray taken to see the break. CFS and mental illness does not work this way. First off, the doctors will go according to the symptoms you are having. They will order the proper test to be done. Once you have gone thru a battery of blood test, x-rays, cat scans and if all of them is normal then the more than likely hood the proper diagnosed is Chronic Fatigue Syndrome. The sad thing right now I know is that the medical field is not taking this illness too seriously. Some doctors just think that you are tired, but it is more than just that. I know my self-years ago, when I first got sick I was bitten by the mosquito that carries the **encephalitis** virus. I was in the hospital for a few weeks for it and was very sick for some time. I was fine for many years but these past few years I was under a lot of stress and I think it weakened my immune system. At first, I had to take frequent naps during the day and after words I felt ok. Then suddenly I was fatigue most part of the day. I would rest many times without getting no relief. It felt as though I did not nap at all. Each day it just got worse. I started to have all sorts of symptoms. I went to the doctor and I told her what I thought it was, so she ordered some tests. They all came out normal. My blood pressure was very high, and I was getting chest pains. I went to the emergency room and was admitted. Once again, I had all sorts of test done. I had a complete heart workup and that was all normal. Finally, being on the right medication my blood pressure came down. I was still having chest pains and very fatigue. After suffering all summer with this I had an upper GI done and it showed that I had a Hiatal Hernia. So, this was the cause of the chest pains. Now we go back to the fatigue. I was seeing a LPN for my depression and she did not change any medications. Finally, I was getting tired of being tired and was getting nowhere. I googled Chronic Fatigue Doctors and found a psychiatrist about an hour from me, so I called and made an appointment. He was very good and thorough. He changed some of my psych medications and I started to feel somewhat better. I was still fatigue during the day time, but it was getting better. See I think not only medical doctors but also psychiatrist should do some studies on CFS. It is very hard to find a good doctor that is up to date on illnesses. Can CFS be both physical and psychological? I say yes. Last year my sister had a heart attack the cause of it was due to stress. She could not afford her apartment, car payment, food and whatever else she needed to live on. So, this started to do damage to her heart, yet all of this was psychological. So, in my case just like her I was under a lot of stress these past few years and it all caught up with me. Since years ago, I had CFS it never left me it just laid dormant until now. So how should the doctors treat me. Well there is much that can be done my new psychiatrist made some changes in my medications and I know when to rest. As I mentioned earlier it is hard somedays. I have to keep a positive outlook that I will once again recover as

I did many years ago, also I look back in the summer

when I first got stricken with this I was a lot worse.  I

am finding I have more energy during the day.

# Chapter 21

## Living a New Life

We all have experienced some type of loss in our lives. Living with CFS is just like a new type of loss. Having Chronic Fatigue Syndrome, we experience loss as losing our past type of living. We have to make adjustments in what we do daily. I know I use to be very active. I liked going to church on Sundays, going walking in parks and anything else out doors. Losing our formal life is just like going thru the grief process as if someone died. In this case, loss of the person we use to be and the person we wanted to become. Grief is usually associated with the death of a loved one, someone we knew, or it can be associated with any other type of loss. If we lose our job, we experience loss is serval ways. We lose our income, perhaps friends we have made on the job. We experience the grieving process of the person we use to be, the things we use to be able to do. I know myself I was very depressed in the beginning because of the type of person I use to be. I realize I now have to deal with the present and hope for the future. I have to make new dreams other that the ones I once had. My dream right now is getting better and hopefully back to the way I once was. We all need to live on faith and hope for if we have faith we can have hope. It is my faith that is getting be thru my illness right now. No matter how bad of a day I have I still rely on my faith to get me thru each day. So, my advice to you is to hold on to your faith no matter how hard of a day you a facing and hope for a better future.

# Chapter 22

## When is it time to exercise?

You must think I am crazy when I say the word exercise. When I say exercise, I mean just do what you can do. Try to walk a little each day. I keep track of my steps each day on my cell phone. The other day I had to do some shopping at Walmart and I wanted to use their electric scooter however there were none available, so I had to walk. I did about 2400 steps for that day and boy did I pay for it. I am feeling a little better however I still feel the fatigue.

When you first start out your exercise therapy you need to figure out your limitations. Exercise is different for a person that has CFS than it is for someone who wants to lose weight. You need to pace yourself and be careful and not to overdo it. If you have a cell phone download an app that counts your steps. Keep track of how many steps you take in one day. If you cannot use an app then just keep track of the time you spend on one exercise. Start out simple and just walk in your house or apartment. Do little steps and take your time. This will also help you relieve stress. If you need to sit down and rest go ahead. To keep your muscles from atrophy you can exercise right in your chair. Lift your legs one at a time for 5 sets on each leg. As time goes by try to increase the sets you do. Next lift your arms one at a time for 5 sets. Now take a rest and increase your sets when you feel ready to.

When you first start out your exercise day start out slow, take frequent rests, and simple moves. One day you may be able to do more than the day before or just the opposite.

Keep a journal of your exercise journey. A very simple tool to use is an exercise log. In the log keep track of the time of day you started to exercise, what you did, how long you exercised for and how you felt after the exercise was over. See a sample of what you may want to do on the next page

| Day/ | Walking | Push | Shoulder | Leg | Wall | Thigh |
|------|---------|------|----------|-----|------|-------|

| Date | | Ups | moves | Lifts | hugger | squeeze |
|---|---|---|---|---|---|---|
| | | | | | | |
| | | | | | | |
| | | | | | | |
| | | | | | | |
| | | | | | | |
| | | | | | | |
| | | | | | | |
| | | | | | | |
| | | | | | | |

You may want to modify your exercise log as you add an exercise to your daily routine. Get plenty of rest after each time you exercise. One day you may be able to do more than the day before. The important thing is to know your limitations.

Below are a few exercises you may want to try:

- Shoulder Moves: Sit in a chair keeping your back straight and feet on the floor. For a count of 5, move your arms up to your shoulders. Just go as far as you can. Hold on a count of 5. Rest for 30 seconds then repeat.

- Leg Lifts: Sit in a chair with your arms holding the sides. Lift the right leg for a count of 5. The goal is to have your leg go straight out, parallel to the floor. Take a rest for 30 seconds then do the same with the left leg. Increase the count as you can. There may be some days where you will not be able to increase but that is ok.

- Wall hugger:  Stand in your doorway.  Using your arm hold the side of the door frame.  Move your body out.  Hold for a count of 12.  Rest for 30 seconds and do another set.

- Thigh Squeeze:  Sit back in your chair.  Place your feet of the floor.  Look straight ahead.  Lift one leg, do a set of 5.  Then switch to the other leg.  As you can increase the sets you do.  Be careful do not over do it.

There are many other exercises for you to do but I think these are good for you to start out with.

Chapter 23

What to avoid if you have CFS

Exercising Beyond Your Capacity. There are some days that you are feeling really good. You start to exercise, and you keep on going beyond your limitations. You do not realize it however once you stop suddenly it catches up with you and now you are at the point that you over did it. This could set you back days or perhaps weeks. When you start an exercise, regimen realize your limitations and do not go beyond that. You will prevent burn out.

Hanging around negative people is not good for anyone not less some who has CFS. The more positive people you associate yourself with the more positive you are going to feel. Sometimes you may have to avoid some of your friends if all they talk about is negative. You will find if you hang out with positive people you will not only start to feel better, but you will start to think positive. If someone tells you, "Ah you are never going to get better," you will tell yourself the same. Where if someone talks about getting better you will start to see that you will start to feel better.

Heaping Meal Portions. We all at one time all another over ate. How about at Thanksgiving Day diner I remember over eating and next thing I was feeling very tired. Having Chronic Fatigue Syndrome alone you feel tired all day not less if you over eat. Over eating is not healthy for anyone. The best advice I can give is to eat just until you feel comfortable. Over eating will do nothing but help you gain weight. The heavier you weigh the more tired you are going to feel.

Partying Past your bedtime is going to do nothing but wear your system down. By not getting the proper rest, you need will catch up with you and make your illness worse. When having an illness like CFS you need to get as much rest as you can. It is not worth staying up past your bedtime and wear your system down. It will take days perhaps weeks to recuperate.

Medicating yourself with alcohol and drugs. First off if you are taking any medications you should not drink at all. It is not good to mix alcohol and medication. It can have an adverse effect and you can end up in a coma. Alcohol is a depressant as it is. This is the last thing you need to add to your body. It will eventually wear your system down and set you back from the progress you have made. Again, I cannot emphasize enough do not mix alcohol with any medications.

Volunteering for over time. You are back to work and feeling great, your boss comes up to you and ask if you can work over time. So sure, you say yes because one you need the money and two you are feeling much better. Well perhaps the first day you will feel ok but if you continue the extra hours of work is going to catch up with your body. Take it easy when you first start back to work. You do not want to take three steps back.

Overtaxing your brain. Take it easy on doing crossword puzzles or other types of games where you have to overtax your brain, or it makes you to think harder. It is good to keep the brain active but once you start to feel tired stop whatever you are doing and rest.

By over working your brain it can tire you out. Best thing to do is do it in moderation. Know what your limitations are.

Under or Overestimating your abilities. What is worse over doing it or not doing enough? Both of them are just as bad as the other. I have to be careful when I am feeling good that I do not over do it. Sometimes when I feel good I just want to keep going. All of a sudden, my system crashes and next thing you know it I am back to the beginning. Lately I start to drive again, and I was feeling pretty good well it caught up with me. It took about two weeks for me to get back to feeling pretty good. However, on the other hand if I do not do anything my muscles will weaken. So, all I did was rest and walked in my apartment. The key thing is to know your limitations and do everything in moderation.

# Chapter 24

## Ways to fight fatigue

Keep your mind busy.  Find something to do that is not

too strenuous.  Make a list of things you need to get

done around the house.  Break your chores up into days

without over doing yourself.  Figure out how long you

can go without having to rest.  Then time yourself as

you go through your day and take break in-between

doing your chores.  By all means do not plan to much in

one day.  If perhaps you cannot finish what you want

to accomplish in that day then just put it on the next

day's list.  The main thing is to keep active.  If you

have dishes that need to be done, you may want to do

just a few at a time then take a break. Then go back to finish doing the dishes. Take this example with anything that you need to do. There are some chores you can do by sitting down. If you can do this then get a chair and sit while doing your chore.

Put down on your list to do a fun time hour. Do anything that you like to do that will not take up too much energy.

Sitting back in your favorite chair. Do not feel guilty if you need to rest. Kick up and relax, watch a good movie, read a good book, listen to music. All of these are a good way to take a break.

Meditation is a good way to relax. I use YouTube videos on guided meditation videos to help me relax. Some nights I will put my head phones on and use these guided meditation videos to help me go to sleep. You

wouldn't believe it however it works.

# Chapter 25

## Meditation and Prayer

Get your mind off your illness by meditation. Prayer helps to build your faith that you will overcome this illness. It only makes you feel stronger. The mind is strong, but the body is weak. By mediating may help ease the panic a fear one finds while having an unknown illness such as CFS. By praying will give you an inner strength. By using the combination of prayer and mediating will help you relax both mind and body. This gives you a chance to get your mind from the negative thoughts you may have in the back of your mind. You may find that your anxiety and chronic pain can disappear for a while.

Below is a step-by-step guide to meditation:

1. Find a comfortable place to either sit or laydown. Turn off your cell phone. Try to make the area nice and dark so you can feel completely at rest.

2. Close your eyes and take three breaths

3. Concentrate on a peaceful place you would like to be at.

4. Get comfortable and try to remain as still as you can. If there are sounds in the air just focus on that peaceful place you are at.

5. When you are ready open your eyes slowly and wake up

6. Try to practice this on a daily basis. Practice it for five minutes then leading up to half an hour.

There are many different mediation videos to watch that are guided. They walk you thru each step to relaxation.

This will help you relax. The relaxation you do not get while you have Chronic Fatigue Syndrome.

Finding ways to keep your mind off your illness can be done. Take for example the step-by-step guide to self-hypnosis. Follow the instructions above on add a favorite place you would like to me as you are meditation. I picture myself at the beach with the sound of the waves in the background. There are Cd's and DVD's that will teach you step by step of self-hypnosis and takes you on a guided imagery journey to a favorite place you would like to be at. It is a good idea to get into practice and do this at least once a day.

# Chapter 26

## Using Herbs and Supplements

Before taking any over the counter medications be sure to check with your doctor.

Below are a few that you may want to try:

- Alpha-lipoic acid: This is a supplement that works as an antioxidant. It fights off "free radicals," or reactive electrons, that attacks your immune system.

- Coenzyme Q10: This is a supplement that may help give you more energy.

- Essential fatty acids (EFA):  This is to help by making your immune system stronger

- Evening primrose oil:  Helps with aches and pains along with giving you more energy.

- Ginseng:  Is used to promote energy and zest.

- Magnesium:  Helps by giving you more energy, build stronger muscles, lift your spirits and aids in your circulation.

- St. John wort:  This is an herb which is a natural antidepressant for some people.

- Vitamin C:  Helps strength your immune system

- Zinc:  This may help with fatigue.

Ask your doctor if you should take any of these and if so how many milligrams.

As with any other medication or vitamins what works for one may not work or the next person.

# Chapter 27

## Handling the Psychological part of CFS

Having any illness can lead to depression. Especially with Chronic Fatigue Syndrome being fatigue and not being able to do things that you once were able to do can and more than likely lead to depression. This does not help your illness. By recognizing the symptoms of depression can help you understand why you are having the symptoms that you are experiencing. This does not mean your illness is all in your head. I know myself I get depressed because my illness does not seem to be getting any better thus leading to hopelessness which is a symptom of depression. Below are just some symptoms you may have which are caused by depression:

- Apathy and lack of enthusiasm

- Crying all the time

- Irritability

- Fatigue

- Feelings of helplessness and hopelessness

- Anxiety

- Loss of concentration

- Insomnia

- Irrational guilt

- Lack of joy in all things

- Lack of self-esteem

- Loss of appetite or eating too much

- Loss of sexual feelings

- Pain

- Suicidal thoughts

- Withdrawal

- Worried or obsessive thoughts.

CFS symptoms are close to that of someone being depressed. Your doctor may want to put you on some medications to help depression. This does not mean you have a mental illness it just helps along with the symptoms you are having. Another good idea is to see a therapist. This will help you talk about your illness. I would suggest finding a therapist that deals with CFS. I see a therapist once a month and it does help me learn how to cope with the illness. It helps to get things off your mind that is bothering you.

# Final Thoughts

I hope this book helped you out. There is a lot more information out there on the internet. Every day doctors and researchers are always finding new ways to treat different illnesses. Hopefully some day they will find a cure or even treatment for CFS.

I cannot stress enough, take one day at a time and somedays one second at a time.

# Credits

The study is published in the journal *PLoS One*

http://www.prohealth.com/me-cfs/me-chronic-fatigue-syndrome-treatment-overview.cfm December 7, 2016 6:03 pm

https://www.bing.com/search?q=ampligen&form=EDGEAR&qs=PF&cvid=ef15194022b346459abff81f29aae990&pq=ampligen December 7, 2016 6:07

https://www.verywell.com/what-is-the-best-treatment-for-chronic-fatigue-syndrome-716068    December   7, 2016

http://www.cdc.gov/cfs/index.html  9/06/2016

http://www.recoveryfromcfs.org/chapter3.htm

The Patient's Guide to Chronic Fatigue Syndrome and Fibromyalgia by Bruce Campbell, Ph. D.

Chronic Fatigue Syndrome for Dummies by Susan R. Lisman, MD and Karla Dougherty

https://medium.com/fatigued-af/10-celebrities-who-have-suffered-from-chronic-fatigue-syndrome-4016fa78b108  1/30/2018 1:47 am

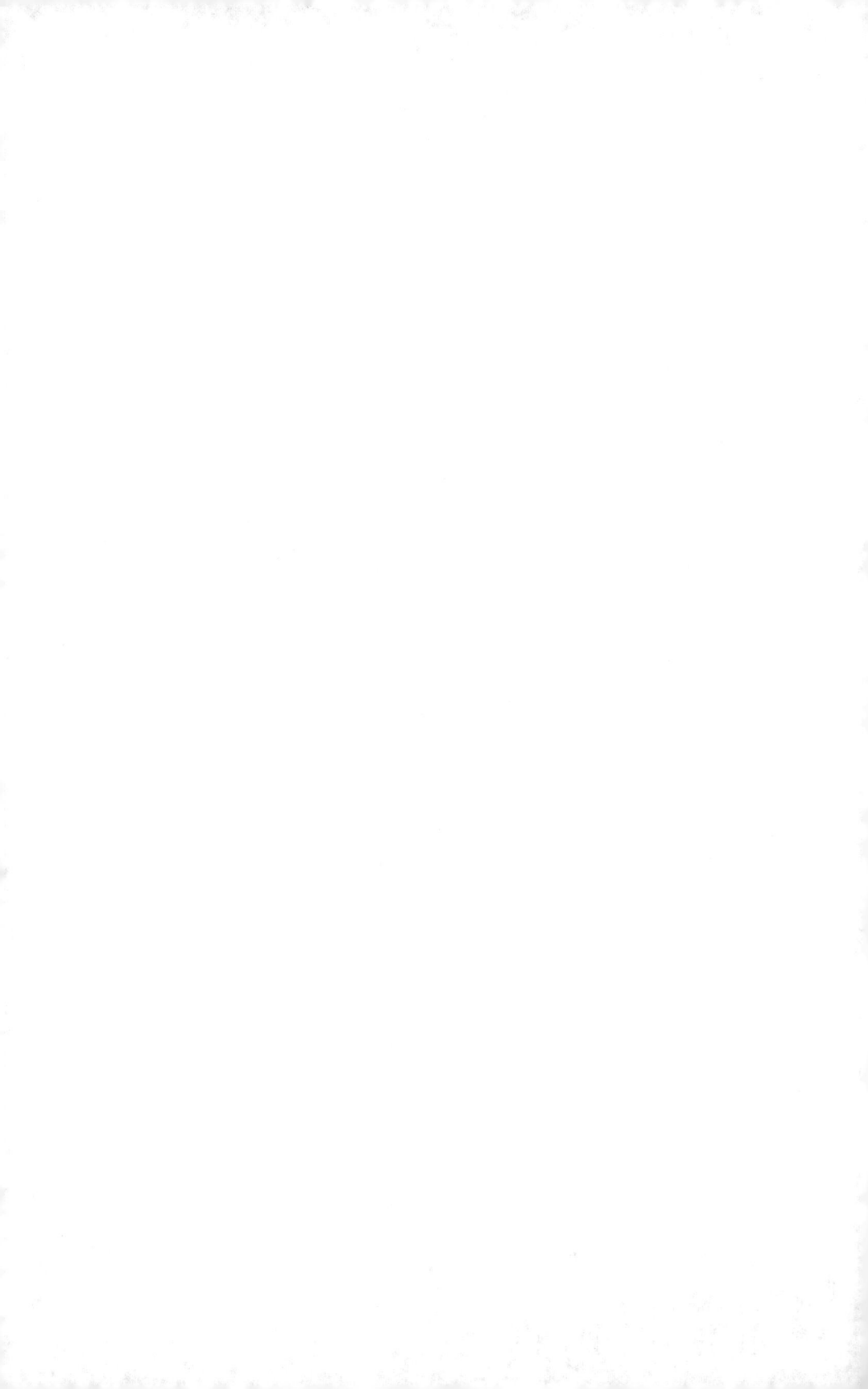